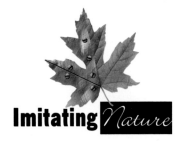

Imitating *Nature*

From BAT SONAR to CANES for the Blind

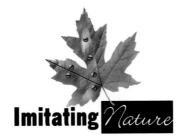

Imitating *Nature*

From BAT SONAR to CANES for the Blind

Toney Allman

KIDHAVEN PRESS
An imprint of Thomson Gale, a part of The Thomson Corporation

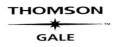

THOMSON

™

GALE

Detroit • New York • San Francisco • San Diego • New Haven, Conn. • Waterville, Maine • London • Munich

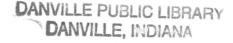

THOMSON

✳ ™

GALE

© 2006 Thomson Gale, a part of The Thomson Corporation.

Thomson and Star Logo are trademarks and Gale and KidHaven Press are registered trademarks used herin under license.

For more information, contact
KidHaven Press
27500 Drake Rd.
Farmington Hills, MI 48331-3535
Or you can visit our Internet site at http://www.gale.com

LIBRARY OF CONGRESS CATALOGING-IN-PUBLICATION DATA

Allman, Toney.
  From bat sonar to canes for the blind / by Toney Allman.
    p. cm. — (Imitating nature)
  Includes bibliographical references and index.
    ISBN 0-7377-3191-5 (hard cover : alk. paper) 1. Canes for the blind—Juvenile literature. 2. Echolocation (Physiology)—Juvenile literature.
  I. Title. II. Series.
  HV1758.A45 2006
  681'.761—dc22
                                                                    2005000729

Printed in The United States of America

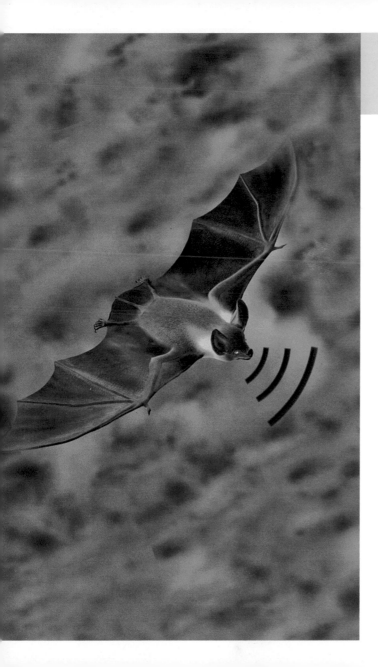

Contents

CHAPTER 1

Seeing with Sound

Dean Waters loves bats—all kinds of bats. He is a **zoologist** and professor at Leeds University in England and an expert in bat behavior. Many bats have an ability that fascinates Waters. They can see with sound. The ability to see with sound is called **echolocation**. Waters thought about how this ability might help people who cannot see. If blind people could imitate echolocation, getting around would be a lot easier for them. But how in the world could people learn to imitate bats? Water's work would eventually lead to an answer.

Bats That See with Sound

Waters studied many kinds of bats. He studied **microbats**, such as the golden-brown Noctules that live in England. Microbats are small, insect-eating bats. There are 750 **species** of microbats living around the world, and all of them can see with sound.

Many bat species find their way around by using their sensitive ears (inset) to detect sound waves bounced off objects.

 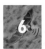

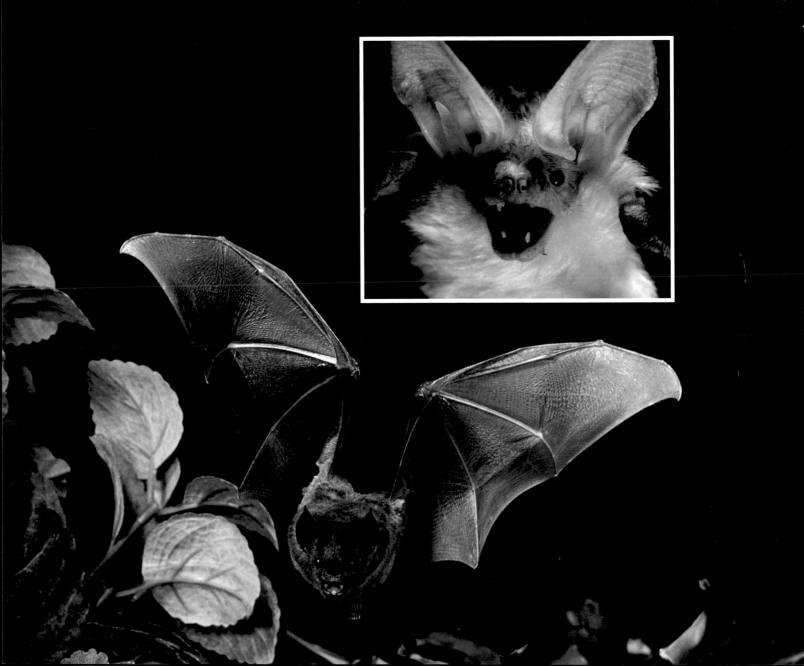

A microbat uses echolocation to find a flower.

Waters also studied Egyptian fruit bats. They are **megabats**, which are large fruit-eating bats that live in warm, tropical places. Some people call them "flying foxes." Of the 162 species of megabats, Egyptian fruit bats are the only ones that can see with sound. Egyptian fruit bats and microbats use echolocation to hunt or fly when it is too dark to see.

How Echolocation Works

While it is flying, a microbat makes high-pitched squeaks, too high for human ears to hear. The high-pitched sounds are called **ultrasound**. Some bats use their noses to make the squeaks; others use their mouths. The squeaks make sound waves that radiate out into the air, like ripples in a lake. When a sound wave hits an object—such as a cave wall, another bat, or an insect—the wave bounces off the object and echoes back to the bat's large, sensitive ears. The strength and speed of the echo tell the bat the nearness and shape of the object ahead.

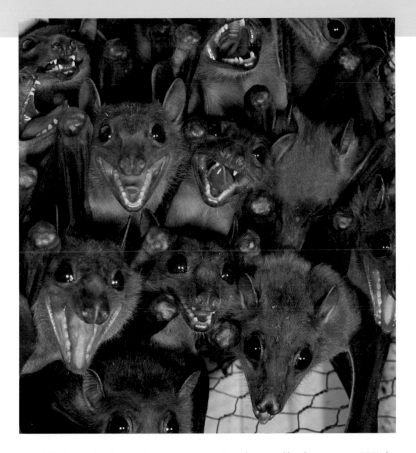

Scientists have invented an electronic device so that people can hear bat squeaks. It is called a bat detector. A bat detector receives ultrasound signals and makes them 32 to 100 times slower than they actually are. This changes the sounds from high pitched to low pitched. So people can then hear the squeaks and chirps of echolocating bats.

Egyptian fruit bats are the only species of megabats that use echolocation to see in the dark.

This echolocation system is also called **sonar**. With it, a microbat speedily wends its way through a black cave. It darts fearlessly in the night sky, avoiding every obstacle and snatching insects from the air. With echolocation, microbats find tons of insects to eat with no trouble.

How Bats Use Echolocation

②

As the sound waves radiate through the air, they reflect off objects back to the bat's sensitive ears, giving the bat a mental picture of its surroundings.

④

When the reflected sound waves become strong enough, the bat zeroes in and snatches its prey out of the air.

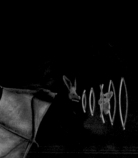

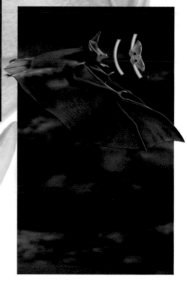

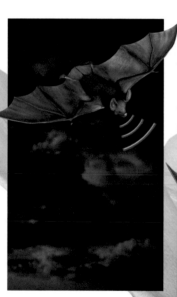

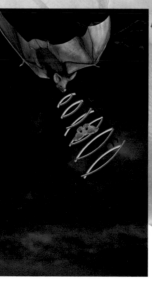

①

A bat sends out squeaks or clicks through its nose or mouth. The squeaks create sound waves, similar to ripples in a lake.

③

By listening to the strength and speed of the sound waves, the bat is able to avoid obstacles and follow its prey.

A Different Kind of Echolocation

Unlike microbats, Egyptian fruit bats make low-pitched sounds to echolocate by clicking their tongues. The clicks bounce off obstacles in front of the bats, just as the high-pitched sounds of microbats do. People can hear the low-pitched clicks of Egyptian fruit bats, so these are not ultrasound. Although this kind of echolocation is not as good at identifying tiny insects as ultrasound is, Egyptian fruit bats use it to avoid obstacles and they never bump into anything.

Making Mental Maps

Whether with ultrasound or clicks, microbats and Egyptian fruit bats use echolocation to find their way in darkness or to hunt for food. The waves of echolocation signals travel through the bats' ears to a special part of their brains. Then their brains translate the signals

Echolocation Wars

Bats use their echolocation ability to home in on prey such as moths and snatch them out of the air. But moths have developed ways of protecting themselves. Some moths can hear echolocation. When they hear an attacking bat, they dive to safety. Other moths can produce ultrasound signals themselves. These signals either startle the bat or jam the bat's echolocation system so that the bat cannot figure out the moth's location, and the moth escapes.

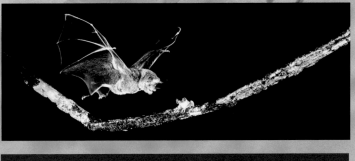

Using echolocation, a frog-eating bat swoops down on a tree frog.

Flashes in the Night

An echolocating bat sends out about ten squeaks per second. So a bat "sees" in fast flashes of ultrasound. A person in the dark who flashes a flashlight off and on as rapidly as possible is seeing somewhat as a bat does.

into mental maps of the bats' surroundings. The mental maps tell the bats where obstacles are and which direction to go to avoid them. The maps are so accurate that bats do not need to use their eyes at all.

People and other animals make mental maps of their surroundings with their brains, too. Their brains use the waves of information signals from eyes and ears to make mental maps. But the human brain has never had any experience with the special sound waves of echolocation.

Could People Do It?

After years of studying bats, Waters had a fascinating question. Could people's brains translate echolocation signals into mental maps of their surroundings? Could they use ultrasound waves just as they use the sound waves that their ears have always been able to hear? The answer to those questions lay a few years in the future. Waters would have to find an easy way to make ultrasound available to human brains. If that were possible, perhaps he could give people who cannot see the power to see with sound.

CHAPTER 2

Echolocation for People

One day in 1998, Waters got together with some friends from Leeds University. Deborah Withington was a specialist in the workings of the human brain. Brian Hoyle was a computer and electronics expert. The three friends chatted about their work, and the talk turned to echolocation. As they shared their knowledge, all three began to get excited about a new idea. They would try inventing an ultrasound echolocation system for people who are blind.

The White Cane for the Blind

Many people who are blind use a long white cane to get from place to place. The cane is swept in front of the person to feel for obstacles in the path. As he or she

A blind artist works on his latest creation. Ultrasound echolocation systems are designed to help him and others like him to get around.

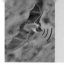

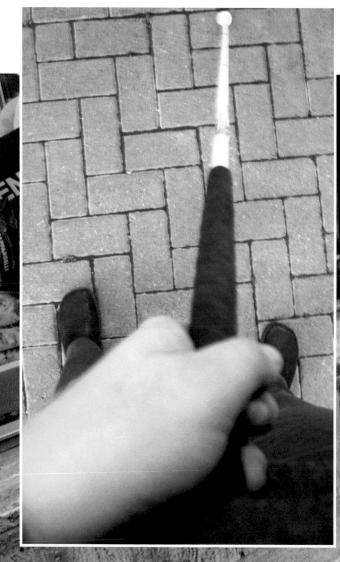

Many blind people use long white canes to locate obstacles in their way as they move from place to place.

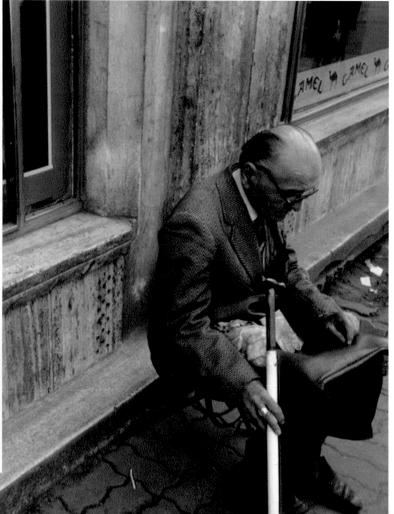

walks along, the cane is moved back and forth and tapped on the ground. If the cane tip knocks into a trash can, for example, then the person knows something is in the way and can walk around it. If the cane touches another person on the sidewalk, the blind person can move to one side and not bump into anyone.

A white cane is very helpful, but it is far from perfect. It gives its user no information about obstacles farther away than the cane tip can reach. It can only be tapped along the ground since swinging a cane in the air would be dangerous to other people or might break things. A cane tells nothing about what may be hanging down at head level, such as a tree branch. It does not warn the user about any object above waist level, such as side-view mirrors on parked cars that stick out into the walkway. It takes a lot of practice and some courage to walk alone with a cane.

Cave Living

Egyptian fruit bats live in black caves and need an echolocation system in order to find their way in the dark. All other megabats roost in trees and are active in the daytime. They never developed echolocation systems because there was no need.

Building a Bat Cane

Waters, Withington, and Hoyle had an idea. What if they attached an echolocation system to a white cane? Then, like a bat, a blind person could see with sound.

Building such an attachment would take knowledge about echolocation, an understanding of human brains, and the ability to develop complicated electronic devices. Waters knew exactly how echolocation worked. Withington knew that people's brains could make mental maps using sight, hearing, and touch. She thought their brains could also understand echolocation, just as bats did. Hoyle believed he could invent an electronic system that mimicked ultrasound echolocation. The three scientists combined their knowledge and got to work.

Transmitters and Sensors

They used a regular white cane but added a special handle. Inside the handle was a small computer connected to four **transmitters**. The transmitters sent out ultrasound signals that bounced off objects and echoed back to the cane. Four **sensors** received the echoes. The sensors were wired to buttons on the cane handle. The buttons changed the ultrasound echoes into vibrations that could be felt with fingers. When a person wrapped his or her hand around the handle, the fingers could feel all four buttons. A button in

How The UltraCane Works

The UltraCane uses echolocation to help blind people avoid obstacles while walking.

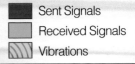

2

Buttons in the handle vibrate when the cane's sensors detect an object is near. The different buttons tell the person where the object is, while the strength of the vibrations indicates how close the object is.

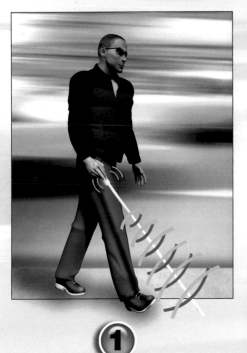

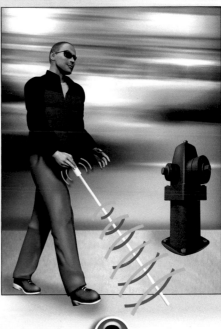

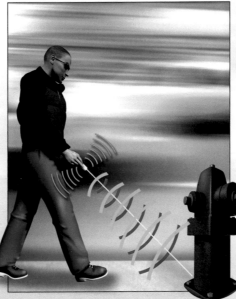

1

The UltraCane's special handle uses transmitters and sensors to send and receive ultrasound signals.

3

By paying close attention to the vibrating buttons, the person is able to change course to avoid obstacles and walk safely.

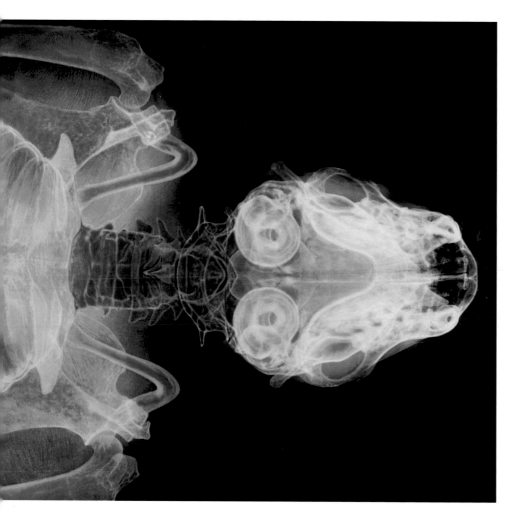

front received ultrasound signals from any object in front of the cane. Two buttons on the back sensed objects on the right and the left. The last button, toward the top of the handle, was set off by objects at head height.

A New Invention

After four years of experiments, the three scientists had an invention they thought would work. They named their invention UltraCane. Like a bat's nose or mouth, it sent ultrasound signals into the air. Like a bat's ears, it also received the signals. But-

An X-ray of a bat skull shows the animal's well-developed inner ears, the organs that make echolocation possible.

tons vibrated whenever the sensors detected an object. The buttons vibrated stronger and faster as the obstacle grew closer. Although the cane could not detect tiny insects as bats can, it could warn of many things in a person's path. The transmitters bounced signals off objects within about 10 feet (3m) of the cane and its user. But now the scientists needed to know if the human brain could translate and understand the signals. The scientists were ready to test their new cane to see if it would work.

Bat Brain Experiments

Dean Waters is doing new experiments with Egyptian fruit bats. He wonders if bat brains can make maps with just one sense and then understand the maps with another sense. For example, if a bat uses echolocation to find its way around a maze, could it follow the same maze with its eyes if its echolocating ability were jammed? When he finds the answer, Waters will know whether bat brains make only one map or if they make two—one for each sense. Someday, this knowledge may help Waters to develop new echolocation inventions for people.

CHAPTER 3

The UltraCane

The first UltraCanes were ready for testing in 2002. The inventors invited a group of blind people to test it out. The testers discovered that using echolocation to "feel" their environment was very easy and comfortable. After a short training period, their brains easily translated the signals vibrating against their fingers. Just like bats' brains, people's brains could make mental maps using ultrasound signals.

Mental Maps

When a car screeches its brakes, a person can instantly turn and look at the source of the sound. The person knows exactly where it came from and where to look. The brain has made a mental map that automatically processes the information signals received from the eyes and ears. Luckily for blind people, ultrasound and touch signals can be used automatically by the brain's mapping system, too.

Lorna Echolocates

One of the first people to test the cane was eleven-year-old Lorna Harvey. Lorna lives in London, England, and has been blind all her life. Lorna did not like the regular white cane. She thought it was difficult to use and looked like something for old people. She did like the UltraCane. She wrapped her hand around the handle so she could feel all four

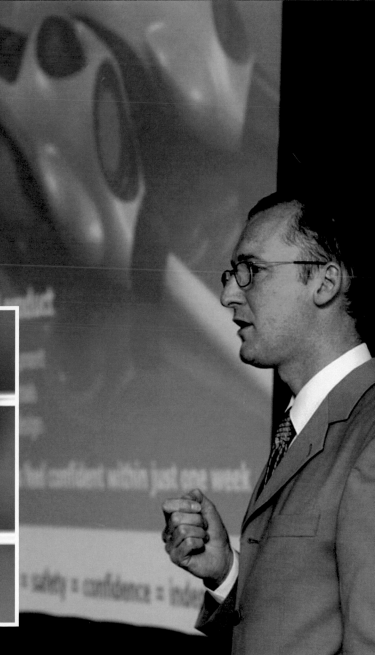

Dean Waters speaks at a conference about the benefits of his UltraCanes (close-up, below) for the blind.

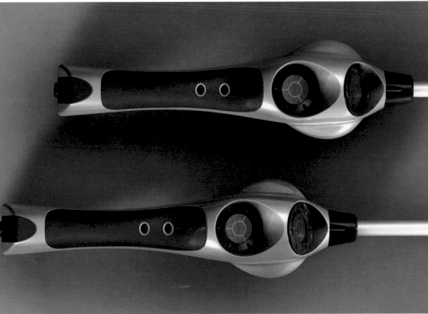

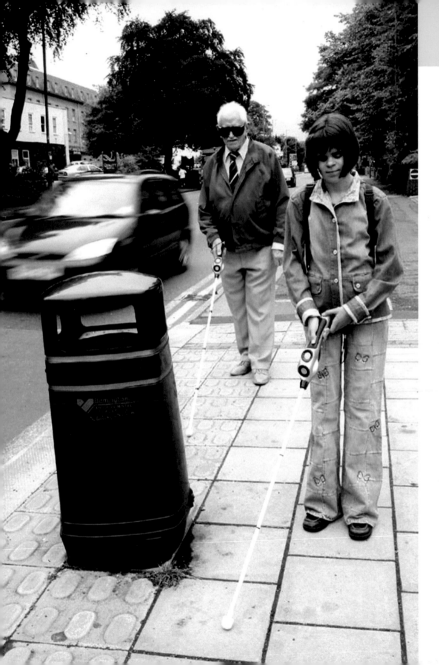

buttons. With her father following closely behind her, she walked all around her neighborhood with the cane.

As Lorna practiced, she learned which vibrating button indicated an obstacle that might be a danger. She could tell by the strength and speed of the vibrations how close she was to an obstacle. She easily moved in a straight line, avoided parked cars, and walked down a crowded alley without her father's help. Lorna even went on television and showed some blind-folded people how to use the echolocating cane.

No More Bumps on the Head

Young people often have an easier time learning new technology than older peo-ple. But older people also easily learned to

Lorna Harvey and an older blind man use the UltraCane to walk safely around the neighborhood.

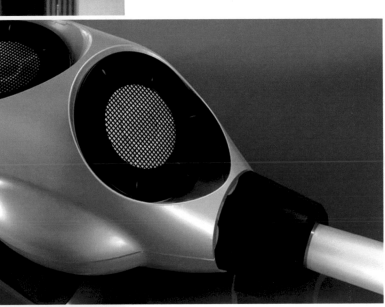

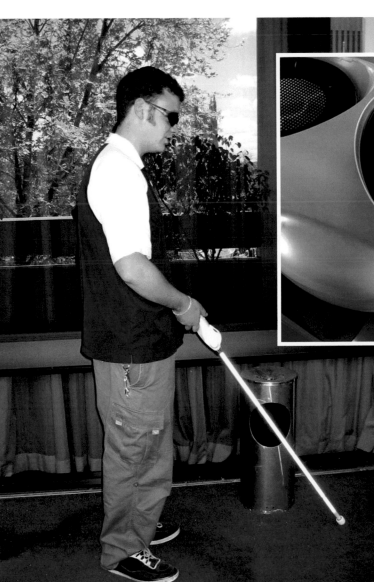

A young blind man walks with the help of an UltraCane. The device's echolocator (inset) can detect objects up to ten feet (3m) away.

use the UltraCane. Peter Vance tried out the UltraCane when it was demonstrated in Australia. Vance hated the way he always bumped his head on low-hanging tree branches when he walked with a regular white cane. With the UltraCane, a button vibrated a warning every time a tree branch loomed in front of him.

Vance loved the freedom he felt when he used echolocation to find his way around. The UltraCane did not find just one obstacle at a time, either. A regular white cane has to touch something before the user knows it is there. The vibrations of the UltraCane revealed a whole map of objects along Vance's route.

Thinking Like a Bat

Roy Gray, another UltraCane tester, liked seeing with sound so much that he refused to give the cane back when the test was over. Gray was 77 years old and had lost most of his sight because of an eye disease eight years earlier. For the first time since he became blind, he was able to walk down the street by himself when he used the UltraCane. He was amazed to discover that following the signals from the buttons felt like a normal, automatic reaction, just as using his eyesight had been in the past.

From Bat Sonar to Canes for the Blind

Another Way to See with Sound

The 'K' Sonar Cane is an echolocation system for the blind invented by Leslie Kay. It is a white cane with an ultrasound handle that is connected to earphones. It beams out ultrasound signals that are reflected back and changed into different tones that can be heard through the earphones. The tones combine into different "tunes" depending on the size and closeness of the obstacle. With practice, a user can learn to recognize the tunes and figure out what objects lie ahead. However, while using the cane and wearing the earphones, the blind person cannot hear other regular sounds, such as traffic noises. This drawback keeps some people from using 'K' Sonar Canes.

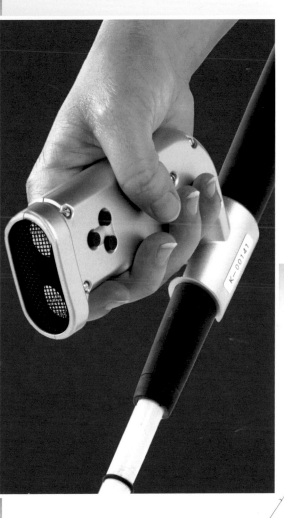

A blind man uses a 'K' Sonar Cane to walk without hitting obstacles.

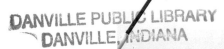

Making Sound Pictures

vOICe is an experimental system for seeing with sound. It was invented by Peter Meijer of the Netherlands. It is a head-mounted camera with headphones and a computer. The camera views the environment and translates everything it sees into sound waves that the user can hear. The numerous sound waves are complicated, but Meijer believes that people's brains can learn to translate these sounds into mental pictures that really let the blind see with their ears. Bright sunshine, for example, is louder than a dim room. Tall objects have a higher sound than short ones. Colors are spoken into the user's ears. Using vOICe is like learning a hard foreign language, but some blind testers have been amazed to discover that their brains actually seem to be seeing the objects that send sounds to them. The letters OIC in vOICe stand for "Oh, I see."

Most people who tested the UltraCane learned to use it comfortably in about one week. Without having to concentrate or think too much, they automatically formed mental maps of their surroundings just as bats did. None of the UltraCane users had to understand the ultrasound technology, practice for a long time, or go to a special school to use the cane. Their fingers and brains easily understood the echolocating vibrations. A new company named Sound Foresight was set up to produce UltraCanes, and in December 2004 it was ready to sell the UltraCane to people everywhere.

Not So Blind After All

There are 180 million people around the world who are blind or who see too poorly to get around on their own. For these people, new ultrasound technology is paving the way to more normal, comfortable, independent lives. Someday, perhaps, ultrasound systems may be only as big as a

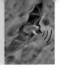

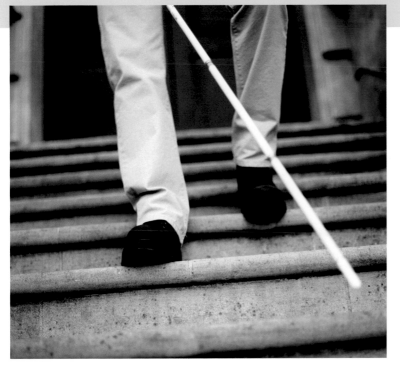

A blind man walks down stairs using a white cane. Echolocating canes help people worldwide to lead independent lives.

cell phone, and a cane might not even be necessary. As the technology improves, echolocating canes may even be able to identify the exact shape, size, and distance of every object in someone's path just as perfectly as bat echolocation can. Then, people's fingers really will be like bats' ears. They will see everything with sound.

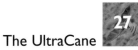

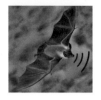

Glossary

echolocation: The way a bat "sees" with its ears, by using reflected sounds to locate and identify objects.

megabats: The 162 species of large bats that usually eat fruit and live in warm, tropical places. Megabats are also called "flying foxes."

microbats: The 750 species of small bats that usually feed on insects and can echolocate.

sensors: Electronic devices that receive signals.

species: A basic category of animals that are closely related and can breed with one another.

transmitters: Electronic devices that produce waves or signals.

ultrasound: Sound that is pitched too high for human ears to hear.

zoologist: A biologist who specializes in the study of animals.

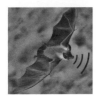

For Further Exploration

Books

Sally Hobart Alexander, *Do You Remember the Color Blue? and Other Questions Kids Ask About Blindness*. New York: Viking, 2000. The author became blind when she was 26 years old. She describes her initial fear and sadness and how eventually she learned to cope without vision. She answers the common questions children ask and includes photographs of her daily life.

Alden R. Carter, *Seeing Things My Way*. Morton, IL: Albert Whitman, 1998. This is an easy-to-read biography of Amanda, a second grader who sees very poorly. With photographs and text, Amanda's day is described with attention to all the normal things she can do despite her disability.

Sandra Markle, *Outside and Inside Bats*. New York: Atheneum Books for Young Readers, 1997. Learn about bat anatomy, bat flight, bat hibernation, and bat echolocation. Plenty of close-up pictures demonstrate the wide variety of bats in the world and their different activities.

Laurence Pringle, *Bats! Strange and Wonderful*. Honesdale, PA: Caroline House, 2000. This easy-to-read book describes bats around the world, the way they live, and what valuable, fascinating creatures they are. It also includes pictures of many different species of bats even vampire bats.

Web Sites

BCI's "Bat Chat" Audiotape (www.batcon.org/discover/echo.html). At this site, you can listen to 3 samples of bat echolocating chirps and squeaks. The ultrasounds have been made audible to human ears with a bat detector.

KidZone Bats (www.kidzone.ws/animals/bats/). This large site has many links with different bat information. See bat photos, play bat games, and learn lots of fun facts about bats.

Questions from Kids about Blindness (www.nfb.org/kids.htm). The National Federation for the Blind has created these pages to answer kids' questions about blindness. Learn about some famous blind people; how blind people read, navigate, work, and attend school, and how they learn to do many things on their own.

Sound Foresight: The UltraCane in Action (www.sound foresight.co.uk/ultracane_demonstrator.htm). Go to this site to see an animated demonstration of a person walking independently with the UltraCane.

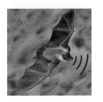

Index

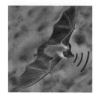

Picture Credits

About the Author

Toney Allman holds degrees from Ohio State University and the University of Hawaii. She currently lives on the Chesapeake Bay in Virginia, where she enjoys sunrises, long walks, and learning about the natural world.